PLANT BASED GUT HEALTH COOKBOOK

Your Essential Cookbook for Easy and Delicious Plant-Based Recipes for a Healthy Gut and Digestive Health.

CHRISTIANA WHITE

GAIN ACCESS TO MORE BOOKS

TABLE OF CONTENTS.

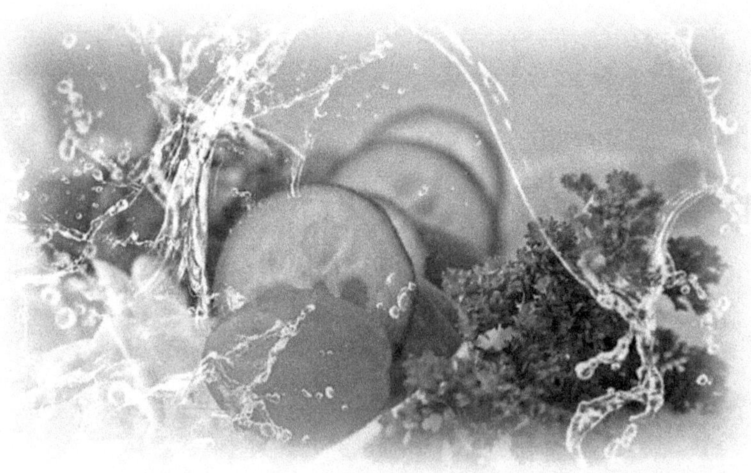

INTRODUCTION

Imagine a life without bloating, gas, constipation, diarrhea, pain, or inflammation in your gut. Imagine yourself energized, cheerful, and confident in your body and mind. Consider eating delicious and healthy plant-based meals that nourish and improve your gut health and wellness.

This isn't a fantasy. This is a reality for many people who follow a plant-based gut health diet. And this might be your reality as well.

Hello, my name is Christiana White, and I'm here to help you alter your gut health and life with a plant-based gut health diet. I have been following a plant-based gut health diet. I've observed directly how this method of eating has helped my digestion, immunity, happiness, and overall health. I've also helped hundreds of folks with gut health issues do the same.

These pages contain more than simply a collection of recipes; they also serve as a roadmap on a life-changing journey toward maximum health. The stories of those who have embarked on this gastronomic adventure are quite motivating.

Consider Mary, who, after years of dealing with digestive issues, found comfort and relief in the healthy meals in these chapters. Imagine John, armed with the information and flavors from this cookbook, saying goodbye to the recurrent ailments that had previously dominated his everyday existence.

This cookbook is more than just a collection of recipes; it demonstrates the transforming power of plant-based living. It's about developing a harmonious relationship with your body, supporting your gut, and embracing the vitality that comes from inside. Through the combination of vivid fruits, strong grains, and nourishing plant-based products, we may enter a world where gut health is cherished rather than regulated.

As you read through these pages, you'll come across a variety of flavors and textures that are intended not just to delight your taste senses but also to nourish your gut bacteria. From the crunch of fresh vegetables in vivid salads to the warmth of soothing stews, each meal is carefully developed, supported by nutritional science, and designed to help you flourish.

Why should you explore the world of plant-based gut health with this cookbook? Because these recipes hold the potential for transformational change. It's more than simply a cookbook; it's a guide on your path to a better, more vibrant you. It's a promise that with each delightful bite, you're nourishing your stomach and planting the seeds of long-term well-being.

By the end of this book, you'll have all the resources and knowledge you need to begin or continue your plant-based gut health journey.

You'll be astounded at how much better you'll feel and look, and how much more you'll appreciate your meals and life.

I'm very excited for you to join me on this journey. I know you'll enjoy this book as much as I did write it for you. I appreciate your confidence and support, and I hope you find this book useful and informative.

So, are you prepared to alter your gut health and your life with a plant-based gut health diet? Let's get started.

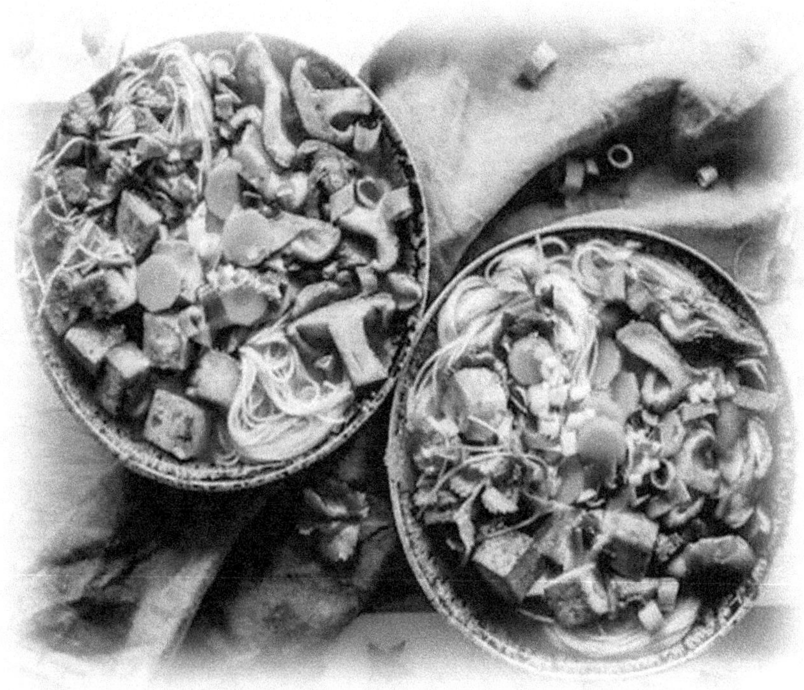

CHAPTER 1

Overview of Plant-Based Gut Health.

Plant-based gut health refers to having a healthy and balanced gut microbiome, which is comprised of trillions of bacteria that live in your digestive tract. These microorganisms, primarily bacteria, play an important role in digestion, immunity, metabolism, mood, and general wellness. They can also increase your risk of getting certain conditions, including obesity, diabetes, cardiovascular disease, and cancer.

A plant-based gut health diet focuses on complete, unprocessed plant foods to nourish and sustain the gut microbiota. These foods include fruits, vegetables, whole grains, legumes, nuts, seeds, and healthy oils. A plant-based gut health diet also restricts or eliminates animal products such as meat, dairy, eggs, and fish, as well as processed foods such refined grains, sugars, oils, and chemicals. These foods can negatively impact the gut microbiome by inducing inflammation, dysbiosis, and leaky gut.

A plant-based gut health diet is not stringent or rigid, but rather flexible and adaptive. You can select the amount of plant-based diet that best fits your interests, needs, and goals. You can also tailor your plant-based gut health diet to your personal and cultural preferences, as well as the availability and cost of foods. The fundamental goal is to consume more plants and less meat, as well as more natural foods and fewer processed foods.

Advantages of a Plant-Based Diet for Gut Health

A plant-based diet can provide numerous benefits to your gut health, including:

• It contains plenty of fibre, which feeds the gut's healthy bacteria and promotes regular bowel motions. Fiber also lowers cholesterol, blood pressure, and blood sugar levels while decreasing the risk of colon cancer.

• It contains a diverse range of phytochemicals, antioxidants, and anti-inflammatory components that protect the gut lining and regulate the immune system. These compounds also serve to reduce oxidative stress, inflammation, and DNA damage, all of which are associated with cancer and other chronic diseases.

• It minimizes consumption of animal products, which might include toxic compounds including antibiotics, hormones, and infections that can upset the intestinal balance. Animal products can also stimulate the synthesis of hazardous metabolites such trimethylamine N-oxide (TMAO), which is linked to cardiovascular disease.

• It aids in the prevention and treatment of common digestive ailments, including irritable bowel syndrome, inflammatory bowel disease, constipation, reflux, and others. People with these diseases may benefit from a plant-based diet since it reduces inflammation, discomfort, bloating, gas, and acid production.

Common Gut Health Issues and Solutions.

People may face the following common gut health issues:

• **Bloating**: A sensation of fullness or swelling in the abdomen, often accompanied by gas and discomfort. Bloating can result from eating too much, too quickly, or too many fermentable carbs, such as beans, onions, garlic, and cruciferous vegetables.

Bloating may also indicate a food intolerance, such as lactose or gluten, or a bacterial overgrowth, such as small intestine bacterial overgrowth (SIBO).

• **Solution**: To prevent or lessen bloating, eat smaller, more frequent meals, chew your food thoroughly, drink plenty of water, avoid carbonated beverages, and restrict or avoid foods that cause bloating.

To aid digestion and reduce bloating, consider consuming probiotics, digestive enzymes, or peppermint oil. If you feel you have a food intolerance or bacterial overgrowth, see your doctor for a diagnosis and treatment.

• **Constipation**: The inability or infrequency of passing stools, which commonly results in hard, dry, or lumpy stools. Constipation can be caused by dehydration, a lack of fibre, inactivity, stress, medicine, or underlying medical disorders like hypothyroidism, diabetes, or Parkinson's disease.

• **Solution**: To prevent or treat constipation, eat more fibre-rich foods including fruits, vegetables, whole grains, and legumes, and drink lots of water. You can also exercise regularly, control your stress, and avoid or restrict constipation-causing foods including dairy, meat, refined carbohydrates, and sugars.

If you require additional assistance, you can try natural laxatives such as prunes, flaxseeds, or psyllium husk, or visit your doctor about prescription or other options.

• **Diarrhea**: Frequent, loose, or watery feces, sometimes accompanied by urgency, cramping, and nausea. Infections, food poisoning, food intolerance, medicine, and inflammatory bowel disease, such as Crohn's or ulcerative colitis, can all induce diarrhea.

• **Solution**: To prevent or treat diarrhea, drink plenty of fluids, particularly water and oral rehydration treatments, to avoid dehydration and electrolyte imbalance. You can also consume bland, easy-to-digest foods like bananas, rice, applesauce, and toast, while avoiding or limiting those that cause diarrhea, such as spicy, fatty, or high-fibre foods.

To restore your gut flora and shorten the duration and intensity of diarrhea, consider taking probiotics, zinc, or anti-diarrheal medicine. If you have signs of illness, such as fever, blood, or mucus in your stools, or if your diarrhea lasts more than a few days, you should consult a doctor.

CHAPTER 2

Essential Ingredients

A plant-based gut health diet comprises complete, unprocessed plant foods that nourish and promote the gut microbiota. These foods include fruits, vegetables, whole grains, legumes, nuts, seeds, and fermented foods.

Each of these food groups delivers different nutrients and benefits for your gut health, including:

• **Whole grains**: These are grains that have not been refined or stripped of the bran, germ, and endosperm, which contain the majority of the fibre, vitamins, minerals, and phytonutrients. Whole grains include oats, barley, buckwheat, quinoa, millet, rye, and others.

They include complex carbohydrates that serve as a source of energy as well as prebiotics for intestinal microbes. They also lower cholesterol, blood sugar, and blood pressure while decreasing the risk of colon cancer.

• **Legumes and pulses**: These are plant seeds from the legume family, which includes beans, peas, lentils, soybeans, chickpeas, and others. They're high in protein, fibre, iron, folate, and other minerals. They also include resistant starch, a carbohydrate that resists digestion and serves as a prebiotic for gut microbes.

They also aid to lower cholesterol, blood sugar, and blood pressure, lowering the risk of cardiovascular disease and diabetes.

• **Fruits and vegetables**: The edible parts of plants include roots, stems, leaves, flowers, and fruits. They include an abundance of vitamins, minerals, antioxidants, and anti-inflammatory substances. They also include numerous types of fibre, including soluble, insoluble, and pectin, which nourish gut microorganisms and support bowel regularity.

They also aid to reduce oxidative stress, inflammation, and DNA damage, all of which are associated with cancer and other chronic diseases.

• **Nuts and seeds**: These are the edible kernels or seeds of plants, including almonds, walnuts, cashews, sunflower seeds, chia seeds, flaxseeds, and others. They include a lot of beneficial fats, like omega-3 and omega-6 fatty acids, which are necessary for the stomach lining and immune system to function properly.

They also supply protein, fibre, magnesium, zinc, and other minerals. They also aid to lower cholesterol, blood sugar, and blood pressure, lowering the risk of cardiovascular disease and diabetes.

• **Fermented foods**: These are foods that have gone through the fermentation process, which involves microorganisms like bacteria, yeast, or fungi converting sugars and starches into alcohol or acids.

Fermented foods include yogurt, kefir, sauerkraut, kimchi, miso, tempeh, and others. Probiotics are living bacteria that can colonize the gut and provide health benefits.

They also create metabolites, such as short-chain fatty acids, that can influence the gut flora and immunological response. They also aid to boost digestion, immunity, mood, and overall health.

These are some of the key elements of a plant-based gut health diet. By incorporating a mix of these items into your regular meals and snacks, you can improve your gut and general health.

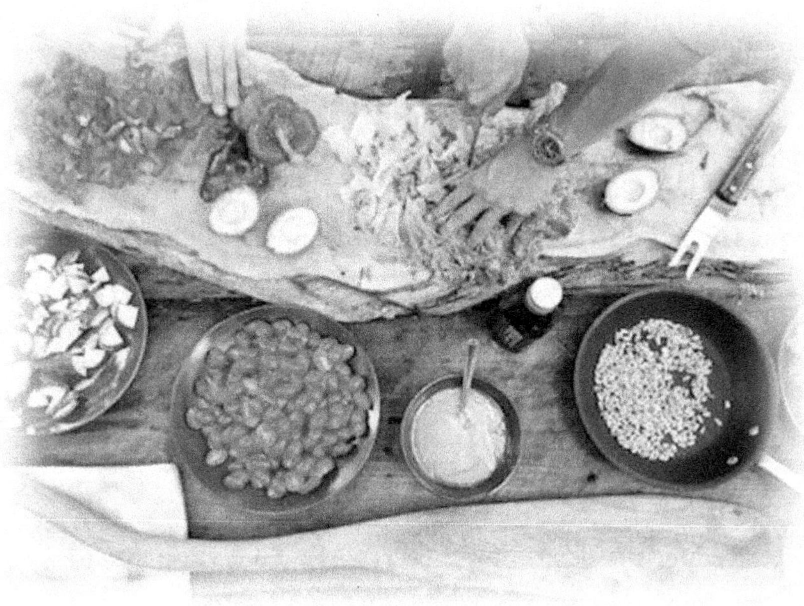

CHAPTER 3

Breakfast Recipes

Oatmeal With Fresh Fruit and Nuts

- _Servings: two._
- _Prep time is 10 minutes._

Ingredients:

- One cup rolled oats.
- Two glasses of water or plant-based milk.
- One pinch of salt.
- 1/4 teaspoon vanilla extract (optional).
- 2 tablespoons maple syrup or another sweetener (optional)
- 1/4 cup chopped nuts (almonds, walnuts, or pecans)
- 1/2 cup of fresh fruits, including apples, bananas, or berries.

Step-by-Step Directions:

- In a small saucepan, cook the oats, water or milk, salt, vanilla, and maple syrup over medium-high heat until boiling.
- Reduce the heat to a simmer, stirring occasionally, for about 15 minutes, or until the oats are soft and creamy.

- Divide the oats between two dishes and top with nuts and berries. Enjoy!

Banana And Peanut Butter Smoothie.

- *Serves: 1*
- *Prepare time: 5 minutes.*

Ingredients:

- One huge ripe banana, peeled and sliced
- 2 tablespoons natural peanut butter.
- 1 cup of plant-based milk (soy, almond, or oat).
- 1/4 teaspoon cinnamon (optional).
- A few ice cubes (optional)

Step-by-Step Directions:

- In a blender, mix the banana, peanut butter, milk, cinnamon, and ice. Blend for approximately 1 minute, or until smooth and frothy.
- Transfer the smoothie to a glass and enjoy!

Avocado Toast with Hummus and Sprouts

- *Servings: two.*
- *Prep time is 10 minutes.*

Ingredients:

- 4 slices whole wheat bread.
- 1/4 cup hummus.
- One ripe avocado, peeled and pitted
- Add salt and pepper to taste.
- 1/4 cup alfalfa sprouts or other microgreens.
- A sprinkle of lemon juice is optional.

Step-by-Step Directions:

- In a toaster or oven, toast the bread for about 5 minutes, or until golden and crisp.
- Spread the hummus equally on the toast slices.
- Mash the avocado with a fork, then season with salt and pepper. Spoon the avocado over the hummus.
- If preferred, sprinkle with lemon juice and top with sprouts. Enjoy!

Scrambled Tofu, Spinach, And Mushrooms

- ***Servings: two.***
- ***Prep time is 20 minutes.***

Ingredients:

- One tablespoon of olive oil.
- 1/4 cup chopped onion.
- 2 garlic cloves, minced
- One cup of sliced mushrooms.
- Two cups baby spinach.
- Add salt and pepper to taste.
- 1 block (14 oz) firm tofu, drained and crumbled
- One-quarter teaspoon of turmeric
- One-quarter teaspoon of cumin
- 1/4 teaspoon paprika.
- Two tablespoons of nutritional yeast.
- Two teaspoons of soy sauce or tamari.
- Optional: a dash of plant-based milk (soy, almond, or oat).

Step-by-Step Directions:

- Warm the oil in a large skillet over medium-high heat. Cook the onion and garlic, stirring regularly, until softened, about 10 minutes.

- Cook, stirring periodically, until the mushrooms are browned and the spinach has wilted, about 10 minutes. Season with salt and pepper, then transfer to a platter. Stay warm.
- In the same skillet, combine the tofu, turmeric, cumin, paprika, nutritional yeast, soy sauce, and milk (if using).
- Cook for about 10 minutes, stirring regularly, until the tofu is thoroughly cooked and coated with the spices.
- Serve the tofu scramble and veggie mixture on two plates and enjoy!

Coconut Yogurt with Granola and Fruit.

- *Servings: two.*
- *Prepare time: 5 minutes.*

Ingredients:

- Two cups plain coconut yogurt.
- One-quarter cup granola
- 1/2 cup fresh berries (strawberries, blueberries, or raspberries)
- 2 tablespoons maple syrup or another sweetener (optional)

Step-by-Step Directions:

- Spoon the coconut yogurt into two bowls and sprinkle with oats.
- Add the berries and drizzle with maple syrup if preferred. Enjoy!

Buckwheat Pancakes Made with Maple Syrup and Almond Butter.

- _**Servings: four.**_
- _**Prep time is 20 minutes.**_

Ingredients:

- 1 cup buckwheat flour.
- One teaspoon of baking powder.
- One pinch of salt.
- 1 cup of plant-based milk (soy, almond, or oat).
- 2 tablespoons maple syrup or another sweetener.
- 2 tablespoons of oil, like olive, canola, or coconut.
- One-quarter cup almond butter
- More maple syrup to serve

Step-by-Step Directions:

- In a large bowl, combine the buckwheat flour, baking powder, and salt.
- In a small bowl, combine the milk, maple syrup, and oil.
- Combine the wet and dry ingredients and stir thoroughly until a smooth batter forms.
- Preheat a lightly greased griddle or skillet over medium-high heat. Drop about 1/4 cup batter onto the griddle and cook for 3 minutes, or until bubbles appear on the surface.
- Cook until the opposite side is browned, which should take around 2 minutes. Repeat with the remaining batter.
- In a small saucepan, boil the almond butter over low heat until smooth and runny, about 5 minutes, stirring regularly.
- Top the pancakes with almond butter and additional maple syrup, if preferred. Enjoy!

Chia Pudding with Mangos and Coconut Milk

- *Servings: two.*
- *Preparation time: 10 minutes, with overnight soak.*

Ingredients:

- 1/4 cup chia seeds.
- One cup coconut milk.

- 2 tablespoons maple syrup or another sweetener.
- 1/4 teaspoon vanilla extract (optional).
- One ripe mango, peeled and diced
- A sprinkle of shredded coconut is optional.

Step-by-Step Directions:

- In a small mixing bowl, combine the chia seeds, coconut milk, maple syrup, and vanilla, if using. Cover and chill overnight, or for at least 4 hours, until the chia seeds have absorbed the liquid and produced a gel-like texture.
- Use a blender to purée half of the mango until smooth and creamy. Set aside.
- Layer the chia pudding and mango puree in two glasses or jars. Optionally, top with the leftover mango pieces and shredded coconut. Enjoy!

Quinoa Porridge with Date and Cinnamon.

- *Servings: two.*
- *Prep time is 20 minutes.*

Ingredients:

- 1 cup quinoa, washed and drained.
- Two glasses of water or plant-based milk.
- One pinch of salt.

- One-fourth teaspoon cinnamon
- 2 tablespoons maple syrup or another sweetener.
- 1/4 cup chopped dates.
- Optional: a dash of plant-based milk (soy, almond, or oat).

Step-by-Step Directions:

- In a small saucepan, cook the quinoa, water or milk, salt, cinnamon, and maple syrup over high heat until boiling. Reduce the heat and simmer, covered, for 15 minutes, or until the quinoa is soft and fluffy.
- Mix in the dates and fluff with a fork.
- Divide the quinoa porridge into two dishes, and add more milk as desired. Enjoy!

Apple and Walnut Muffins

- *Serves: 12*
- *Prepare time: 30 minutes.*

Ingredients:

- Two cups of whole wheat flour.
- One teaspoon of baking soda.
- A half teaspoon of salt.
- 1/4 teaspoon nutmeg.
- One-quarter teaspoon of cloves

- 1/4 cup oil (coconut, canola, or olive)
- 1/2 cup maple syrup or another sweetener.
- 1/4 cup plant-based milk (soy, almond, or oat)
- 1/4 cup unsweetened applesauce.
- One teaspoon of vanilla extract.
- 1 cup grated apple.
- 1/2 cup chopped walnuts.

Step-by-Step Directions:

- Preheat the oven to 180°C (350°F) and prepare a 12-cup muffin pan with paper liners or cooking spray.
- In a large bowl, combine the flour, baking soda, salt, nutmeg, and cloves.
- In a small mixing bowl, combine the oil, maple syrup, milk, applesauce, and vanilla.
- Combine the wet and dry ingredients and stir thoroughly until a smooth batter forms.
- Fold in the apples and walnuts.
- Spoon the batter into the prepared muffin cups, about 3/4 full.
- Bake for 18–20 minutes, or until a toothpick inserted in the center comes out clean.
- Allow the muffins to cool briefly in the pan before transferring to a wire rack to cool entirely.

- Enjoy!

<u>Vegetable And Bean Burritos</u>

- ***Servings: four.***
- ***Prepare time: 30 minutes.***

Ingredients:

- One tablespoon of olive oil.
- 1/4 cup chopped onion.
- 2 garlic cloves, minced
- One teaspoon of cumin.
- One-half teaspoon of chili powder
- One-quarter teaspoon of salt
- 1/4 teaspoon black pepper.
- 1 cup cooked black beans (drained and rinsed)
- One-quarter cup salsa
- Four whole wheat tortillas.
- 1/4 cup shredded vegan cheese (optional).
- 1/4 cup chopped lettuce.
- 1/4 cup chopped tomatoes.
- 2 tablespoons vegan sour cream (optional).
- 2 tablespoons chopped cilantro (optional).

Step-by-Step Directions:

- Warm the oil in a large skillet over medium-high heat. Cook the onion and garlic, stirring regularly, until softened, about 10 minutes.
- Cook for 10 minutes, stirring regularly, until the cumin, chili powder, salt, pepper, beans, and salsa are thoroughly heated.
- Heat the tortillas in the microwave or oven for about 10 seconds, or until soft and flexible.
- Spread about 1/4 of the bean mixture in the center of each tortilla. If using, sprinkle with cheese. Fold the bottom edge over the filling, then fold in the sides and roll tight.
- Divide the burritos in half and garnish with lettuce, tomato, sour cream, and cilantro if preferred. Enjoy!

CHAPTER 4

Lunch Recipes

Lentil And Vegetable Soup.

- ***Servings: four.***
- ***Prep time is 40 minutes.***

Ingredients:

- One tablespoon of olive oil.
- 1 onion, chopped
- Two carrots, peeled and chopped
- Two celery stalks, diced
- 2 garlic cloves, minced
- One teaspoon dried thyme.
- One teaspoon of dried rosemary.
- Add salt and pepper to taste.
- Four cups of veggie broth.
- Two glasses of water.
- Rinse and drain 1 cup of brown or green lentils.
- Two bay leaves.
- Two cups of chopped kale or spinach.
- Two teaspoons of lemon juice.

- Fresh parsley for garnish (optional).

Step-by-Step Directions:

- In a big pot, heat the oil to medium-high heat. Cook the onion, carrots, celery, garlic, thyme, rosemary, salt, and pepper, stirring periodically, until the onion is tender, about 15 minutes.
- Bring the broth, water, lentils, and bay leaves to a boil. Reduce the heat and cover until the lentils are cooked, which should take around 20 minutes.
- Add the kale or spinach and lemon juice, and simmer for 5 minutes, or until the greens wilt.
- Remove the bay leaves and spoon the soup into bowls. Garnish with parsley if desired. Enjoy!

Chickpea And Kale Salad with Tahini Dressing.

- *Servings: four.*
- *Prep time is 20 minutes.*

Ingredients:

• For the Salad:

- 4 cups of chopped kale with stems removed.
- Two teaspoons of lemon juice.

- Add salt and pepper to taste.

- 2 cups cooked chickpeas, drained and rinsed.

- 1/4 cup chopped red onion.

- 1/4 cup chopped fresh parsley.

- Two teaspoons of sunflower seeds.

• *For dressing:*

- 1/4 cup tahini.

- Two teaspoons of water.

- Two teaspoons of lemon juice.

- One garlic clove, minced

- Add salt and pepper to taste.

Step-by-Step Directions:

- In a large bowl, massage the lemon juice, salt, and pepper into the kale until soft and wilted, about 10 minutes.

- Toss together the chickpeas, onion, parsley, and sunflower seeds.

- In a small bowl, combine the tahini, water, lemon juice, garlic, salt, and pepper. Whisk until smooth and creamy.

- Drizzle dressing over salad and toss to combine. Enjoy!

Roasted Veggie and Hummus Wrap

- *Servings: four.*
- *Prep time is 40 minutes.*

Ingredients:

• *For roasted vegetables:*

- One-quarter cup olive oil
- Two teaspoons of balsamic vinegar.
- Add salt and pepper to taste.
- 1 zucchini, sliced
- One yellow squash, sliced
- One red bell pepper, sliced
- One red onion, sliced

• *For wrapping:*

- Four whole wheat tortillas.
- 1/2 cup hummus.
- Four lettuce leaves.
- 1/4 cup chopped fresh basil.

Step-by-Step Directions:

- Preheat the oven to 200 °C (400 °F) and line a baking sheet with parchment paper.
- In a small bowl, combine the oil, vinegar, salt, and pepper.

- Place the zucchini, squash, bell pepper, and onion on the prepared baking sheet, then sprinkle with the oil mixture. Toss to coat and spread into an equal coating.
- Roast the vegetables for 25-30 minutes, or until soft and browned, flipping halfway through.
- Heat the tortillas in the microwave or oven for about 10 seconds, or until soft and flexible.
- Spread 2 tablespoons hummus on each tortilla, then top with a lettuce leaf and a quarter of the roasted vegetables. Sprinkle with basil and roll tightly.
- Slice the wraps in half and enjoy!

Black Bean and Corn Quinoa Dish.

- ***Servings: four.***
- ***Prepare time: 30 minutes.***

Ingredients:

- 1 cup quinoa, washed and drained.
- Two cups of veggie broth or water.
- Add salt and pepper to taste.
- 1 tablespoon olive, canola, or coconut oil.
- 1/4 cup chopped onion.
- 2 garlic cloves, minced

- One teaspoon of cumin.

- 1/4 teaspoon smoked paprika.

- 1/4 teaspoon oregano.

- One-quarter teaspoon of chili powder

- One-quarter teaspoon of salt

- 1/4 teaspoon black pepper.

- One (15 oz) can of black beans, drained and rinsed

- One cup of fresh or frozen corn kernels.

- 1/4 cup chopped fresh cilantro.

- Two teaspoons of lime juice.

- One peeled and sliced avocado

- One-quarter cup salsa

Step-by-Step Directions:

- Heat the quinoa, broth or water, salt, and pepper in a small saucepan over high heat until boiling.

- Reduce the heat to a simmer and cover for 15 to 20 minutes, or until the quinoa is frothy and the liquid has been absorbed. Fluff with a fork, then set aside.

- Warm the oil in a large skillet over medium-high heat. Cook the onion and garlic, stirring regularly, until softened, about 10 minutes.

- Cook for about 10 minutes, stirring regularly, until the cumin, smoked paprika, oregano, chili powder, salt, pepper, beans, and corn are thoroughly heated.
- Stir in the cilantro and lime juice, then remove from heat.
- Divide the quinoa into four bowls, then top with the bean and corn combination, avocado, and salsa. Enjoy!

Spicy Tofu and Broccoli Stir-Fry

- ***Servings: four.***
- ***Prep time is 25 minutes.***

Ingredients:

- One block (14 ounces) of firm tofu, drained and pressed
- Two teaspoons of cornstarch.
- Add salt and pepper to taste.
- Two tablespoons of oil, like coconut, canola, or sesame.
- Four cups of broccoli florets.
- One-quarter cup water
- Two teaspoons of soy sauce or tamari.
- 2 tablespoons maple syrup or another sweetener.
- 1 tablespoon of sriracha or another hot sauce.
- One teaspoon of grated ginger.
- 2 garlic cloves, minced

- Two teaspoons of sesame seeds.
- 2 tablespoons chopped scallions.
- Cooked rice to serve

Step-by-Step Directions:

- Cut the tofu into bite-sized pieces and combine with the cornstarch, salt, and pepper in a big Ziplock bag or mixing bowl.
- Heat oil in a big skillet over high heat. Cook the tofu, stirring regularly, until golden and crisp on all sides, about 15 minutes. Transfer to a dish to keep heated.
- In the same skillet, combine the broccoli and water and heat until boiling. Cover and steam for approximately 5 minutes, or until the broccoli is bright green and crisp-tender. Drain then return to the skillet.
- In a small mixing bowl, combine the soy sauce, maple syrup, sriracha, ginger, and garlic. Toss the broccoli and tofu with the sauce. Cook for approximately 5 minutes, or until the sauce has thickened slightly.
- Garnish with sesame seeds and scallions, then serve with rice. Enjoy!

Mushroom And Spinach Risotto

- _**Servings: four.**_
- _**Prep time is 40 minutes.**_

Ingredients:

- Four cups of veggie broth.
- 2 tablespoons of oil, like olive, canola, or coconut.
- 1/4 cup chopped onion.
- 2 garlic cloves, minced
- 1 1/2 cups arborio rice.
- 1/4 cup of white wine or more broth
- Add salt and pepper to taste.
- Two cups of sliced mushrooms.
- Two cups baby spinach.
- One-quarter cup nutritional yeast
- Two tablespoons of vegan butter.
- Fresh parsley for garnish (optional).

Step-by-Step Directions:

- In a small saucepan, bring the broth to a boil over high heat. Reduce the heat to stay warm.
- Warm the oil in a large skillet over medium-high heat. Cook the onion and garlic, stirring regularly, until softened, about 10 minutes.

- Toast the rice, stirring regularly, for about 5 minutes, or until it is slightly brown.

- Pour in the wine or broth and simmer, stirring frequently, for about 2 minutes, until absorbed.

- Pour in the broth one ladle at a time, stirring constantly and allowing for each addition to be absorbed before adding the next, until the rice is creamy and al dente, about 20 to 25 minutes. Season with salt and pepper to taste.

- Cook until the mushrooms are soft and the spinach has wilted, about 10 minutes.

- Add the nutritional yeast and vegan butter, and mix thoroughly.

- Garnish with parsley if desired, and enjoy!

Creamy Cauliflower and Potato Curry.

- ***Servings: four.***
- ***Prep time is 35 minutes.***

Ingredients:

- 1 tablespoon olive, canola, or coconut oil.

- 1 onion, chopped

- 3 garlic cloves, minced

- One tablespoon of grated ginger.

- Two teaspoons of curry powder.

- One teaspoon of turmeric.

- 1/2 teaspoon cumin.

- One-quarter teaspoon of salt

- 1/4 teaspoon black pepper.

- One (14-ounce) can of coconut milk

- Two cups of veggie broth.

- 4 cups chopped cauliflower.

- Two cups diced potatoes.

- Two teaspoons of cornstarch.

- Two teaspoons of water.

- Fresh cilantro for garnish (optional).

Step-by-Step Directions:

- In a big pot, heat the oil to medium-high heat. Cook the onion, garlic, ginger, curry powder, turmeric, cumin, salt, and pepper for about 15 minutes, stirring regularly, until the onion is tender.

- Bring the coconut milk and broth to a boil. Add the cauliflower and potatoes, then reduce the heat to a simmer and cover for about 15 minutes, or until cooked.

- In a small mixing basin, combine the cornstarch and water. Whisk until smooth. Stir into the curry and heat, stirring, until the sauce thickens, about 5 minutes.

- Serve with cilantro, if desired, and enjoy!

Vegetable And Bean Chili

- ***Servings: six.***
- ***Prep time is 40 minutes.***

Ingredients:

- 1 tablespoon olive, canola, or coconut oil.
- 1 onion, chopped
- One green bell pepper, chopped
- Two carrots, peeled and chopped
- Two celery stalks, diced
- 4 garlic cloves, minced
- Two tablespoons of chili powder.
- One tablespoon of cumin.
- One teaspoon of oregano.
- 1/2 teaspoons of smoked paprika.
- One-quarter teaspoon of salt
- 1/4 teaspoon black pepper.
- One (28-ounce) can of crushed tomatoes.
- Two cups of veggie broth.
- One (15 oz) can of black beans, drained and rinsed
- One (15-ounce) can of kidney beans, drained and rinsed

- One (15-ounce) can of drained corn

- Two teaspoons of apple cider vinegar.

- Serve with vegan cheese, sour cream, and onions (optional).

Step-by-Step Directions:

- In a big pot, heat the oil to medium-high heat. Cook the onion, bell pepper, carrots, celery, garlic, chili powder, cumin, oregano, smoked paprika, salt, and pepper, stirring occasionally, until the onion is tender, about 15 minutes.

- Bring the tomatoes, broth, beans, and corn to a boil. Reduce the heat and let the chili to simmer, uncovered, for about 20 minutes, or until thick and flavorful.

- Stir in the vinegar and taste, adjusting the spice as needed.

- Optional toppings include vegan cheese, sour cream, and scallions. Enjoy!

Mediterranean Couscous Served with Olives and Sun-Dried Tomatoes

- *Servings: four.*
- *Prep time is 20 minutes.*

Ingredients:

- 1 1/2 cups veggie broth.

- 1 cup couscous.

- Add salt and pepper to taste.

- 1/4 cup chopped fresh parsley.

- Two teaspoons of lemon juice.

- 2 tablespoons of oil (olive or sunflower)

- 1/4 cup sliced olives (kalamata or green)

- 1/4 cup chopped sun-dried tomatoes.

- 2 teaspoons of drained capers.

- Two tablespoons of roasted pine nuts.

Step-by-Step Directions:

- In a small saucepan, bring the broth to a boil over high heat. Add the couscous, salt, and pepper, and toss. Remove from heat and cover with a lid.

- Allow to rest for 10 minutes, or until the couscous is fluffy and the liquid is absorbed. Fluff with a fork before transferring to a large bowl.

- Toss together the parsley, lemon juice, oil, olives, sun-dried tomatoes, capers, and pine nuts.

- Enjoy either heated or cold!

Tomato And Basil Spaghetti.

- ***Servings: four.***
- ***Prep time is 25 minutes.***

Ingredients:

- 12 ounces of whole wheat pasta, including spaghetti, penne, or fusilli.
- Add salt and pepper to taste.
- Two tablespoons of olive or canola oil.
- 4 garlic cloves, minced
- 1/4 teaspoon red pepper flakes (optional).
- 4 cups cherry tomatoes (halved)
- A quarter cup of veggie broth or water
- Two teaspoons of balsamic vinegar.
- 1/4 cup chopped fresh basil.
- Vegan parmesan cheese to serve (optional)

Step-by-Step Directions:

- Cook the pasta in a large pot of boiling salted water until al dente, as directed on the package. Drain and return to the pot.
- Warm the oil in a large skillet over medium-high heat. Stir in the garlic and red pepper flakes, if using, and simmer for about 1 minute, or until fragrant.

- Bring the tomatoes, broth/water, vinegar, salt, and pepper to a boil. Reduce the heat to a simmer, stirring occasionally, for about 15 minutes, or until the tomatoes are mushy and the sauce has thickened somewhat.
- Stir in the basil and taste, adjusting the spice as needed.
- Top the spaghetti with tomato sauce and vegan parmesan cheese, if desired. Enjoy!

CHAPTER 5

<u>*Dinner Recipes*</u>

<u>*Sweet Potato and Black Bean Burgers.*</u>

- ***Servings: four.***
- ***Prep time is 40 minutes.***

Ingredients:

- Two medium sweet potatoes, peeled and diced
- 2 tablespoons of oil, like olive, canola, or coconut.
- Add salt and pepper to taste.
- One (15 oz) can of black beans, drained and rinsed
- A quarter cup of oat flour or breadcrumbs
- 2 teaspoons smoked paprika.
- One teaspoon of cumin.
- One-quarter teaspoon of garlic powder
- Four whole wheat hamburger buns.
- Serve with lettuce, tomato, onion, avocado, and vegan mayonnaise (optional).

Step-by-Step Directions:

- Preheat the oven to 200 °C (400 °F) and line a baking sheet with parchment paper.

- In a large bowl, combine the sweet potatoes, 1 tablespoon oil, salt, and pepper. Spread them evenly on the prepared baking sheet and roast for 25 to 30 minutes, or until soft and golden, tossing once halfway through.
- In a food processor, combine the black beans, oat flour, smoked paprika, cumin, garlic powder, salt, and pepper until a coarse texture forms. Transfer to a large bowl and mash with a fork or potato masher.
- Add the roasted sweet potatoes and mash again until thoroughly mixed. Shape the mixture into four patties and arrange them on the same baking pan.
- Brush with the remaining oil and bake for 15 to 20 minutes, or until firm and golden. Flip halfway through.
- In a toaster or oven, toast the burger buns for about 5 minutes, or until gently crisp.
- Build the burgers with the buns, patties, and toppings of your choosing. Enjoy!

Vegetable And Tofu Lasagna.

- *Serves: 8*
- *Prep time is 60 minutes.*

Ingredients:

• For the Tofu Ricotta:

- One block (14 ounces) of firm tofu, drained and pressed
- One-quarter cup nutritional yeast
- Two teaspoons of lemon juice.
- Two teaspoons of olive oil.
- 2 garlic cloves, minced
- Add salt and pepper to taste.

• For veggie sauce:

- Two tablespoons of olive or canola oil.
- 1 onion, chopped
- Two carrots, peeled and chopped
- Two celery stalks, diced
- 2 zucchini, diced
- 4 garlic cloves, minced
- One teaspoon of dried oregano.
- One teaspoon dried basil.
- Add salt and pepper to taste.
- One (28-ounce) can of crushed tomatoes.

- Two cups of veggie broth.
- Two tablespoons of tomato paste.
- Two bay leaves.

• *For lasagna:*

- Twelve no-boil lasagna noodles.
- 2 cups vegan mozzarella cheese, shredded
- Fresh basil to garnish (optional)

Step-by-Step Directions:

- Crumble the tofu into a large bowl, then mix in the nutritional yeast, lemon juice, oil, garlic, salt, and pepper. Mash with a fork or potato masher until well incorporated and smooth. Set aside.
- Heat the oil in a big pot over medium-high heat. Cook the onion, carrots, celery, zucchini, garlic, oregano, basil, salt, and pepper, stirring periodically, until the onion is translucent, about 15 minutes.
- Bring the tomatoes, broth, tomato paste, and bay leaves to a boil. Reduce the heat and let the sauce simmer, uncovered, for about 20 minutes, or until thick and delicious. Discard the bay leaves, then taste and adjust the spice as needed.
- Heat the oven to 180°C (350°F) and lightly butter a 9x13-inch baking dish.

- To assemble the lasagna, apply a thin layer of vegetable sauce on the bottom of the prepared baking dish. Place four noodles over the sauce, slightly overlapping.

- Spread half of the tofu ricotta over the noodles, then add a third of the veggie sauce and cheese. Add another layer of noodles, tofu ricotta, vegetable sauce, and cheese. Garnish with the leftover noodles, veggie sauce, and cheese.

- Cover the baking dish with foil and bake for 25-30 minutes, or until the noodles are soft and the cheese has melted.

- Allow the lasagna to rest for ten minutes before slicing and serving. Garnish with basil if desired. Enjoy!

Mushroom And Lentil Shepherd's Pie.

- ***Servings: six.***
- ***Prep time is 50 minutes.***

Ingredients:

• *For potato topping:*

- 4 big peeled and diced potatoes.
- Add salt and pepper to taste.
- 1/4 cup plant-based milk (soy, almond, or oat)
- Two tablespoons of vegan butter.
- Two tablespoons of nutritional yeast.

• *For the mushroom-lentil filling*

- Two tablespoons of olive or canola oil.

- 1 onion, chopped

- 4 garlic cloves, minced

- Four cups of sliced mushrooms.

- Two teaspoons dried thyme.

- Two teaspoons of dried rosemary.

- Add salt and pepper to taste.

- Two teaspoons of soy sauce or tamari.

- Two teaspoons of cornstarch.

- Two cups of veggie broth.

- 2 cups cooked brown or green lentils, drained and rinsed.

- One cup frozen pea.

- Fresh parsley for garnish (optional).

Step-by-Step Directions:

- Heat the oven to 180°C (350°F) and lightly butter a 9x13-inch baking dish.

- To make the potato topping, cook the potatoes in a large saucepan of salted water until soft, about 15 to 20 minutes. Drain and return to the pot. Mash together the milk, butter, nutritional yeast, salt, and pepper until smooth and creamy. Set aside.

- Preheat the oil in a large skillet over medium-high heat. Cook the onion, garlic, mushrooms, thyme, rosemary, salt, and pepper for about 15 minutes, turning periodically, until the onion is tender and the mushrooms are browned.
- In a small bowl, combine the soy sauce, cornstarch, and broth. Whisk until smooth. Pour in the mushroom mixture and bring to a boil. Reduce the heat to a simmer and stir until the sauce thickens, about 10 minutes.
- Stir in the lentils and peas, then remove from heat.
- To make the shepherd's pie, evenly distribute the mushroom and lentil mixture in the prepared baking dish. Spoon the potato mixture over the filling and gently spread to cover it thoroughly.
- Bake for 25–30 minutes, or until the potato topping is brown and the filling is bubbling.
- Garnish with parsley if desired, and enjoy!

Thai Green Curry with Rice

- *Servings: four.*
- *Prep time is 25 minutes.*

Ingredients:

- 2 cups jasmine rice.
- Four cups of water.
- Salt to taste.
- 1 tablespoon oil, such as coconut, canola, or sesame.
- One-quarter cup green curry paste
- One (14-ounce) can of coconut milk
- 2 tablespoons of brown sugar (or another sweetener)
- Two teaspoons of lime juice.
- Two cups of chopped broccoli.
- One red bell pepper, sliced
- One cup of sliced bamboo shoots.
- 1/4 cup chopped fresh basil.
- Fresh cilantro for garnish (optional).

Step-by-Step Directions:

- In a small saucepan, bring the rice, water, and salt to a boil on high heat. Reduce the heat to a simmer and cover for 15 to 20 minutes, or until the rice is cooked and the water has been absorbed. Fluff with a fork and stay warm.

- Warm the oil in a large skillet over medium-high heat. Stir in the curry paste and heat for 1 minute, or until aromatic.
- Bring the coconut milk, sugar, lime juice, and salt to a boil. Reduce the heat to a simmer and whisk until slightly thickened, about 10 minutes.
- Stir in the broccoli, bell pepper, and bamboo shoots and simmer for about 10 minutes, or until the veggies are crisp tender.
- Stir in the basil and taste, adjusting the spice as needed.
- Serve the curry over rice, garnished with cilantro if desired. Enjoy!

Moroccan Tagine with Couscous

- *Servings: four.*
- *Prep time is 40 minutes.*

Ingredients:

• For the Tagine:

- Two tablespoons of olive or canola oil.
- 1 onion, chopped
- 4 garlic cloves, minced
- One teaspoon ground cumin
- One teaspoon of ground coriander.

- One teaspoon of ground cinnamon.

- 1/2 teaspoon ground turmeric.

- One-quarter teaspoon of salt

- 1/4 teaspoon black pepper.

- One (14-ounce) can of diced tomatoes.

- Two cups of veggie broth.

- 2 cups diced butternut squash.

- Two cups of diced carrots.

- One (15 oz) can of drained and washed chickpeas

- 1/4 cup chopped dried apricots.

- 2 teaspoons of freshly chopped parsley.

- 2 teaspoons of chopped fresh cilantro.

• *For the Couscous:*

- 1 1/2 cups veggie broth.

- 1 cup couscous.

- Add salt and pepper to taste.

- 2 tablespoons of oil (olive or sunflower)

- Two teaspoons of lemon juice.

- 2 teaspoons of chopped fresh mint.

Step-by-Step Directions:

- Preheat the oil in a big pot over medium-high heat. Cook the onion, garlic, cumin, coriander, cinnamon, turmeric, salt, and pepper, stirring periodically, until the onion is tender, about 15 minutes.

- Bring the tomatoes, broth, squash, carrots, chickpeas, and apricots to a boil. Reduce the heat and cover, simmering for about 20 minutes, or until the vegetables are soft.

- Stir in the parsley and cilantro, taste, and adjust seasoning as needed.

- To prepare the couscous, bring the broth to a boil in a small saucepan over high heat. Add the couscous, salt, and pepper, and toss.

- Remove from heat and cover with a lid. Allow to rest for 10 minutes, or until the couscous is fluffy and the liquid is absorbed. Fluff with a fork, then stir in the oil, lemon juice, and mint.

- Serve the tagine with couscous and enjoy!

Eggplant And Chickpea Moussaka

- *Servings: six.*
- *Prep time is 60 minutes.*

Ingredients:

• *For the eggplant and chickpea layers:*

- Two large eggplants, sliced

- Add salt and pepper to taste.

- Two tablespoons of olive or canola oil.

- 1 onion, chopped

- 4 garlic cloves, minced

- One teaspoon of dried oregano.

- 1/2 teaspoon cinnamon.

- 1/4 teaspoon nutmeg.

- One-quarter teaspoon of salt

- 1/4 teaspoon black pepper.

- One (28-ounce) can of crushed tomatoes.

- 2 cups cooked chickpeas, drained and rinsed.

- 2 teaspoons of freshly chopped parsley.

- *Prepare the béchamel sauce:*

  - One-quarter cup vegan butter

  - 1/4 cup all-purpose flour.

  - 3 cups of plant-based milk (soy, almond, or oat).

  - Add salt and pepper to taste.

  - A pinch of nutmeg.

  - One-quarter cup nutritional yeast

Step-by-Step Directions:

- Heat the oven to 180°C (350°F) and lightly butter a 9x13-inch baking dish.

- Sprinkle the eggplant slices with salt and let them sit in a strainer for 15 minutes to remove excess moisture. Rinse, then pat dry with paper towels.

- Place the eggplant slices in a single layer on two baking pans and brush with oil. Bake for 15 to 20 minutes, or until brown and tender. Flip halfway through.

- Warm the oil in a large skillet over medium-high heat. Cook the onion, garlic, oregano, cinnamon, nutmeg, salt, and pepper, stirring periodically, until the onion is tender, about 15 minutes.

- Bring the tomatoes, chickpeas, and parsley to a boil. Reduce the heat to a simmer, stirring regularly, for about 20 minutes, or until the sauce is thick and delicious.

- To make the béchamel sauce, melt the butter in a small saucepan over medium heat. Stir in the flour and simmer for about 2 minutes, or until smooth and bubbling.

- Bring the milk, salt, pepper, and nutmeg to a boil, whisking in gradually. Reduce the heat to a simmer and stir until the sauce is thick and creamy, about 10 minutes. Stir in the nutritional yeast and remove from heat.

- To build the moussaka, spread a thin layer of the tomato and chickpea mixture in the prepared baking dish. Spread half of the eggplant slices over the sauce, slightly overlapping.

- Spread half of the béchamel sauce over the eggplant, carefully covering it thoroughly. Repeat with the remaining tomato-chickpea mixture, eggplant slices, and béchamel sauce.

- Bake for 25–30 minutes, or until the sauce is bubbling and golden.

- Allow the moussaka to rest for 10 minutes before slicing and serving. Enjoy!

Tempeh and Vegetable Skewers

- *Servings: four.*
- *Prep time is 35 minutes (including marinating time).*

Ingredients:

• *For marinade:*

- 1/4 cup soy sauce (or tamari)
- 2 tablespoons maple syrup or another sweetener.
- Two tablespoons of oil, like coconut, canola, or sesame.
- Two teaspoons of apple cider vinegar.
- 2 garlic cloves, minced
- One teaspoon of grated ginger.
- 1/4 teaspoon red pepper flakes (optional).

• **For skewers:**

- 1 block (8 oz) tempeh, sliced into bite-sized cubes.

- Two cups cherry tomatoes.

- Two cups of button mushrooms.

- 1 green bell pepper chopped into bits.

- 1 red onion, chopped into bits

- Add salt and pepper to taste.

- Fresh parsley for garnish (optional).

Step-by-Step Directions:

- In a small mixing bowl, combine the soy sauce, maple syrup, oil, vinegar, garlic, ginger, and red pepper flakes (if using).

- Place the tempeh cubes in a big Ziplock bag or shallow dish, then pour the marinade over them. Seal or cover and chill for at least 2 hours, or up to overnight, turning occasionally to coat.

- Preheat the oven to 200 °C (400 °F) and line a baking sheet with parchment paper. Alternatively, grill the skewers over medium-high heat for 15 minutes, rotating regularly, until browned and cooked through.

- Thread the tempeh and vegetables onto wooden or metal skewers, alternating them as desired.

- Sprinkle with salt and pepper and place on the prepared baking sheet. Save the remaining marinade for basting.

- Bake for 20-25 minutes, or until the tempeh is browned and the vegetables are soft, basting halfway through with the marinade.
- Garnish with parsley if desired, and enjoy!

Lentil And Walnut Loaves

- *Serves: 8*
- *Prep time is 60 minutes.*

Ingredients:

- Two tablespoons of olive or canola oil.
- 1 onion, chopped
- Two carrots, peeled and grated
- Two celery stalks, diced
- 4 garlic cloves, minced
- Two teaspoons dried thyme.
- Two teaspoons of dried sage.
- Add salt and pepper to taste.
- 2 cups cooked brown or green lentils, drained and rinsed.
- 1 cup of roasted and chopped walnuts.
- A quarter cup of oat flour or breadcrumbs
- 2 tablespoons of ground flaxseed.
- One-quarter cup water

- Two teaspoons of soy sauce or tamari.

- Two tablespoons of ketchup.

• *For glaze:*

- 1/4 cup ketchup.

- 2 tablespoons maple syrup or another sweetener.

- One tablespoon of apple cider vinegar.

- One teaspoon of smoked paprika.

- One pinch of salt.

Step-by-Step Directions:

- Heat the oven to 180°C (350°F) and lightly butter a 9x5-inch loaf pan.

- Warm the oil in a large skillet over medium-high heat. Cook the onion, carrots, celery, garlic, thyme, sage, salt, and pepper, stirring periodically, until the onion is translucent, about 15 minutes.

- In a food processor, combine the lentils, walnuts, oat flour, flaxseeds, water, soy sauce, and ketchup until a coarse texture forms. Transfer to a large mixing bowl and combine thoroughly.

- Press the mixture firmly into the prepared loaf pan, smoothing the surface. Bake 25 minutes, or until firm and lightly browned.

- To prepare the glaze, combine the ketchup, maple syrup, vinegar, smoked paprika, and salt in a small mixing dish.

- Spread the glaze evenly over the loaf and bake for an additional 10 minutes, or until bubbling and caramelized.

- Allow the bread to rest for ten minutes before slicing and serving. Enjoy!

Cauliflower And Almond Cheese Pizza

- ***Servings: four.***
- ***Prep time is 40 minutes.***

Ingredients:

• *For the crust:*

- Four cups of cauliflower florets.
- One-quarter cup almond flour
- 2 tablespoons of ground flaxseed.
- Two teaspoons of water.
- Add salt and pepper to taste.
- One-quarter teaspoon of garlic powder
- 1/4 teaspoon oregano.

• *Regarding the cheese:*

- 1/4 cup raw almonds, soak for at least 4 hours or overnight.

- One-quarter cup water

- Two tablespoons of nutritional yeast.

- One tablespoon of lemon juice.

- Add salt and pepper to taste.

- *For toppings:*

- One-quarter cup pizza sauce

- 1/4 cup sliced olives.

- 1/4 cup sliced mushrooms.

- 2 teaspoons of freshly chopped basil.

Step-by-Step Directions:

- Preheat the oven to 200 °C (400 °F) and line a baking sheet with parchment paper.

- Using a food processor, pulse the cauliflower until it resembles rice. Transfer to a microwave-safe bowl and cook for 5 minutes, or until softened.

- Allow it cool somewhat before squeezing out the excess moisture with a cheesecloth or clean kitchen towel.

- In a small dish, whisk together the flaxseeds and water and set aside for 10 minutes, or until thick and gel-like.

- In a large bowl, combine the cauliflower, almond flour, flax mixture, salt, and pepper.

CHAPTER 6

Snack and Dessert Recipes

Carrot And Apple Cake

- *Serves: 12*
- *Prep time is 50 minutes.*

Ingredients:

- Two cups of whole wheat flour.
- 2 tablespoons baking powder.
- One-half teaspoon of baking soda
- A half teaspoon of salt.
- One teaspoon of cinnamon.
- 1/4 teaspoon nutmeg.
- One-quarter teaspoon of cloves
- 1/4 cup oil (coconut, canola, or olive)
- 1/2 cup maple syrup or another sweetener.
- 1/4 cup plant-based milk (soy, almond, or oat)
- 1/4 cup unsweetened applesauce.
- One teaspoon of vanilla extract.
- 1 1/2 cups shredded carrot.
- 1 cup grated apple.
- 1/2 cup chopped walnuts.

- ***For frosting:***

  - 1/4 cup vegan butter, softened

  - 1/4 cup softened vegan cream cheese.

  - Two cups powdered sugar.

  - One teaspoon of vanilla extract.

Step-by-Step Directions:

- Heat the oven to 180°C (350°F) and gently butter a 9x13-inch baking pan.

- In a large mixing bowl, combine the flour, baking powder, soda, salt, cinnamon, nutmeg, and cloves.

- In a small mixing bowl, combine the oil, maple syrup, milk, applesauce, and vanilla.

- Combine the wet and dry ingredients and stir thoroughly until a smooth batter forms.

- Fold in the carrots, apples, and walnuts.

- Pour the batter into the prepared pan, spreading it evenly. Bake for 25–30 minutes, or until a toothpick inserted in the center comes out clean.

- Allow the cake to completely cool in the pan before icing.

- Using an electric mixer, combine the butter and cream cheese to create the frosting smooth and creamy. Gradually add the powdered sugar and vanilla, beating until frothy and smooth.

- Spread the icing on the cake and cut it into twelve pieces. Enjoy!

Chocolate And Peanut Butter Brownies.

- *Serves: 16*
- *Prep time is 40 minutes.*

Ingredients:

• *Regarding the brownies:*

- 1/4 cup oil (coconut, canola, or olive)
- 1/4 cup plant-based milk (soy, almond, or oat)
- 1/4 cup maple syrup or another sweetener.
- One teaspoon of vanilla extract.
- One cup oat flour.
- One-quarter cup cocoa powder
- A half teaspoon of baking powder.
- One-quarter teaspoon of salt
- 1/4 cup vegan chocolate chips.

• *Directions for the peanut butter swirl:*

- 1/4 cup natural peanut butter.
- 2 tablespoons maple syrup or another sweetener.
- 1 tablespoon of plant-based milk (soy, almond, or oat)

Step-by-Step Directions:

- Preheat the oven to 180°C (350°F) and prepare an 8x8-inch baking tray with parchment paper.

- In a large mixing bowl, combine the oil, milk, maple syrup, and vanilla until thoroughly blended.

- In a small bowl, combine the oat flour, cocoa powder, baking powder, and salt.

- Combine the dry ingredients with the wet components and mix thoroughly until a thick batter forms. Stir in the chocolate chips.

- Pour the batter into the prepared pan, spreading it evenly.

- In a small mixing bowl, combine the peanut butter, maple syrup, and milk until smooth and creamy.

- Drop dollops of the peanut butter mixture onto the brownie batter and swirl with a knife or toothpick to create a marbled pattern.

- Bake for 20–25 minutes, or until a toothpick inserted in the center comes out largely clean.

- Allow the brownies to completely cool in the pan before cutting into 16 squares. Enjoy!

Oat and Raisin Cookies

- *Servings: 24.*
- *Prep time is 25 minutes.*

Ingredients:

- 1/4 cup oil (coconut, canola, or olive)
- 1/4 cup plant-based milk (soy, almond, or oat)
- 1/4 cup maple syrup or another sweetener.
- One teaspoon of vanilla extract.
- 1 1/2 cups rolled oats.
- One cup of whole wheat flour.
- One-half teaspoon of baking soda
- One-quarter teaspoon of salt
- One-fourth teaspoon cinnamon
- 1/2 cup raisins.

Step-by-Step Directions:

- Preheat the oven to 180°C (350°F), then line two baking sheets with parchment paper.
- In a large mixing bowl, combine the oil, milk, maple syrup, and vanilla until thoroughly blended.
- In a small basin, combine the oats, flour, baking soda, salt, and cinnamon.

- Combine the dry and wet ingredients and stir thoroughly until a sticky dough forms. Stir in the raisins.
- Drop by rounded tablespoonfuls onto the prepared baking sheets, leaving enough space between each. Flatten slightly with your fingers or a spatula.
- Bake for 10–12 minutes, or until brown and hard around the edges.
- Allow the cookies to cool briefly on the baking sheets before moving them to a wire rack to cool entirely. Enjoy!

Banana and Oat Bars

- *Serves: 12*
- *Prepare time: 30 minutes.*

Ingredients:

- 3 ripe bananas (mashed)
- 1/4 cup oil (coconut, canola, or olive)
- 1/4 cup maple syrup or another sweetener.
- One teaspoon of vanilla extract.
- Two cups rolled oats.
- 1/4 cup chopped walnuts.
- 1/4 cup vegan chocolate chips.
- One-quarter teaspoon of salt

Step-by-Step Directions:

- Heat the oven to 180°C (350°F) and gently butter a 9x9-inch baking pan.
- In a large mixing bowl, blend the bananas, oil, maple syrup, and vanilla until thoroughly incorporated.
- Combine the oats, walnuts, chocolate chips, and salt, stirring until a thick dough forms.
- Spread the batter evenly in the prepared pan and smooth the top.
- Bake for 18–20 minutes, or until brown and firm.
- Allow the bars to cool completely in the pan before cutting into twelve pieces. Enjoy!

Kale Chips

- ***Servings: four.***
- ***Prepare time: 15 minutes.***

Ingredients:

- One bunch of washed and dried kale
- 1 tablespoon oil, such as olive or coconut.
- Add salt and pepper to taste.
- Two tablespoons of nutritional yeast.

Step-by-Step Directions:

- Preheat the oven to 180°C (350°F), then line two baking sheets with parchment paper.
- Tear the kale leaves into bite-sized pieces, discarding the stems. Toss in a large basin with the oil, salt, and pepper until evenly coated.
- Spread the kale in a single layer on the prepared baking pans, then sprinkle with nutritional yeast.
- Bake for 10-15 minutes, or until crisp and brown, rotating halfway through.
- Enjoy as a snack or side dish!

Apple And Almond Butter Slices.

- *Servings: two.*
- *Prepare time: 5 minutes.*

Ingredients:

- One large apple, cored and sliced
- Two tablespoons of natural almond butter.
- One-fourth teaspoon cinnamon
- One pinch of salt.

Step-by-Step Directions:

- Place the apple slices on a big plate or platter.
- Heat the almond butter in a small microwave-safe bowl for 10 to 15 seconds, or until it's runny.
- Drizzle almond butter over the apple slices, then sprinkle with cinnamon and salt.
- Enjoy as a snack or dessert!

Date and Nut Balls

- *Serves: 16*
- *Prepare time: 15 minutes.*

Ingredients:

- One cup of pitted dates.
- 1/2 cup raw almonds.
- 1/4 cup raw cashews.
- Two tablespoons of cocoa powder.
- One-quarter teaspoon of salt
- One-quarter teaspoon of vanilla extract
- Optional: shredded coconut for coating.

Step-by-Step Directions:

- Using a food processor, pulse the dates until they form a sticky paste. Transfer to a big bowl and set aside.
- In the same food processor, pulse the almonds and cashews until finely chopped. Add the cocoa powder, salt, and vanilla, and pulse to combine.
- Combine the nut mixture and date paste, and mix well with your hands until a dough forms.
- Divide the dough into 16 balls and, if desired, roll in shredded coconut. Refrigerate for at least an hour until firm. Enjoy!

Fruit and Nut Trail Mix

- ***Serves: 8***
- ***Prepare time: 5 minutes.***

Ingredients:

- One cup raw almond.
- 1/2 cup raw pistachios.
- One-quarter cup pumpkin seeds
- One-quarter cup sunflower seeds
- 1/4 cup dried cranberries.
- One-quarter cup dried cherries

- 1/4 cup dried apricots, chopped

- One-quarter cup dark chocolate chips

Step-by-Step Directions:

- In a large mixing bowl, combine the almonds, pistachios, pumpkin seeds, sunflower seeds, cranberries, cherries, apricots, and chocolate chips until well combined.

- Keep the trail mix in an airtight container or Ziplock bag at room temperature or in the fridge for up to a month. Enjoy!

Popcorn Containing Nutritional Yeast and Spices

- *Servings: four.*
- *Prep time is 10 minutes.*

Ingredients:

- 1/4 cup popcorn kernels.
- 2 tablespoons of oil, like olive, canola, or coconut.
- Add salt and pepper to taste.
- Two tablespoons of nutritional yeast.
- One-half teaspoon of garlic powder
- One-half teaspoon of onion powder
- 1/4 teaspoon paprika.

Step-by-Step Directions:

- In a large lidded pot, heat the oil over medium-high heat. Add the popcorn kernels and seal with the lid. Shake the pot occasionally to keep the kernels from burning.
- Cook for 5 to 7 minutes, or until the popping sound has subsided. Remove from the heat and place the popcorn in a large bowl.
- Toss with salt, pepper, nutritional yeast, garlic powder, onion powder, and paprika until evenly coated. Enjoy!

Roasted Chickpeas

- *Servings: four.*
- *Prep time is 25 minutes.*

Ingredients:

- Two (15-ounce) cans of drained and rinsed chickpeas
- Two tablespoons of olive or canola oil.
- Add salt and pepper to taste.
- Two teaspoons of cumin.
- One teaspoon of smoked paprika.
- 1/4 teaspoon cayenne pepper (optional).

Step-by-Step Directions:

- Preheat the oven to 200 °C (400 °F) and line a baking sheet with parchment paper.
- Using paper towels, dry the chickpeas and transfer them to a large bowl. Toss in the oil, salt, pepper, cumin, smoked paprika, and cayenne pepper (if using) until evenly coated.
- Place the chickpeas in a single layer on the prepared baking sheet and bake for 15 to 20 minutes, or until crisp and golden, shaking the pan halfway through.
- Great as a snack or salad topping!

CHAPTER 7

Smoothie Recipes

Green Smoothie Containing Spinach, Banana, And Almond Milk

- _Serves: 1_
- _Prepare time: 5 minutes._

Ingredients:

- One cup of fresh spinach.
- One ripe banana, peeled and sliced
- One cup of unsweetened almond milk.

Step-by-Step Directions:

- In a blender, mix the spinach, banana, and almond milk. Blend until smooth and creamy, adding additional milk as needed to adjust consistency.
- Pour in a glass and enjoy!

Berry Smoothie Made with Blueberries, Strawberries, And Soy Milk.

- *Serves: 1*
- *Prepare time: 5 minutes.*

Ingredients:

- 1/2 cup frozen blueberries.
- One-half cup frozen strawberries
- One cup unsweetened soy milk.

Step-by-Step Directions:

- In a blender, mix the blueberries, strawberries, and soy milk. Blend until smooth and frothy, adding additional milk as needed to adjust consistency.
- Pour in a glass and enjoy!

Tropical Smoothie Containing Pineapple, Mango, And Coconut Water

- *Serves: 1*
- *Prepare time: 5 minutes.*

Ingredients:

- 1/2 cup frozen pineapple chunks.
- 1/2 cup frozen mango chunks.
- One cup of coconut water.

Step-by-Step Directions:

- In a blender, mix the pineapple, mango, and coconut water. Blend until smooth and refreshing, adding water as needed to adjust consistency.
- Pour in a glass and enjoy!

Chocolate Smoothie Containing Cocoa, Banana, And Oat Milk

- *Serves: 1*
- *Prepare time: 5 minutes.*

Ingredients:

- One ripe banana, peeled and sliced
- Two tablespoons of cocoa powder.
- One cup unsweetened oat milk.

Step-by-Step Directions:

- In a blender, mix the banana, cocoa powder, and oat milk. Blend until smooth and chocolaty, adding milk as needed to adjust consistency.
- Pour in a glass and enjoy!

<u>*Golden Smoothie Containing Turmeric, Ginger, And Orange Juice*</u>

- *Serves: 1*
- *Prepare time: 5 minutes.*

Ingredients:

- One-quarter teaspoon of turmeric powder
- One-quarter teaspoon of ginger powder
- One cup of fresh orange juice.

Step-by-Step Directions:

- In a blender, mix the turmeric, ginger, and orange juice. Blend until smooth and bright, adding juice as needed to adjust consistency.
- Pour in a glass and enjoy!

14-Day Meal Plan

Day 1

- Breakfast is oatmeal with fresh fruits and nuts.
- Lunch is lentil and vegetable soup.
- Dinner is sweet potato and black bean burgers.
- Snack: Carrot and apple cake.
- Green smoothie made with spinach, banana, and almond milk.

Day 2

- Breakfast: A banana and peanut butter smoothie.
- Lunch: Chickpea and Kale Salad with Tahini Dressing
- Dinner: vegetable and tofu lasagna.
- Snack: Chocolate and peanut butter brownies.
- Smoothie: Berry smoothie made with blueberries, strawberries, and soy milk

Day 3

- Breakfast: Avocado toast, hummus, and sprouts.
- Lunch: roasted vegetables and hummus wrap.
- Dinner is mushroom and lentil shepherd's pie.
- Snack: oatmeal and raisin cookies

- Tropical smoothie made with pineapple, mango, and coconut water.

Day 4

- Breakfast: scrambled tofu with spinach and mushrooms.
- Lunch: A black bean and corn quinoa bowl.
- Dinner: Thai green curry and rice.
- Snack: Banana and oatmeal bars.
- Chocolate smoothie made with cocoa, banana, and oat milk.

Day 5

- Breakfast: Coconut yogurt with granola and berries.
- Lunch: Spicy tofu and broccoli stir-fry.
- Dinner: Moroccan tagine and couscous.
- Snack: Date and Nut Balls
- Smoothie: Golden smoothie containing turmeric, ginger, and orange juice

Day 6

- Breakfast is buckwheat pancakes with maple syrup and almond butter.
- Lunch is mushroom and spinach risotto.
- Dinner is stuffed peppers with quinoa and beans.
- Snack: Fruit and Nut Trail Mix

- Green smoothie made with spinach, banana, and almond milk.

Day 7

- Breakfast is chia pudding with mango and coconut milk.
- Lunch: A creamy cauliflower and potato curry.
- Dinner is eggplant and chickpea moussaka.
- Snack: popcorn seasoned with nutritional yeast and spices
- Smoothie: Berry smoothie made with blueberries, strawberries, and soy milk

Day 8

- Breakfast: quinoa porridge with dates and cinnamon.
- Lunch: Vegetable and Bean Chili
- Dinner: Tempeh and vegetable skewers.
- Snack: Roasted Chickpeas
- Tropical smoothie made with pineapple, mango, and coconut water.

Day 9

- Breakfast: Apple and Walnut Muffins
- Lunch is Mediterranean couscous with olives and sun-dried tomatoes.
- Dinner: lentil and walnut loaf.
- Snack: Kale Chips.

- Chocolate smoothie made with cocoa, banana, and oat milk.

Day 10

- Breakfast is oatmeal with fresh fruits and nuts.
- Lunch: Tomato and Basil Pasta
- Dinner is cauliflower and almond cheese pizza.
- Snack: Carrot and apple cake.
- Smoothie: Golden smoothie containing turmeric, ginger, and orange juice

Day 11

- Breakfast: A banana and peanut butter smoothie.
- Lunch is lentil and vegetable soup.
- Dinner is sweet potato and black bean burgers.
- Snack: Chocolate and peanut butter brownies.
- Green smoothie made with spinach, banana, and almond milk.

Day 12

- Breakfast: Avocado toast, hummus, and sprouts.
- Lunch: Chickpea and Kale Salad with Tahini Dressing
- Dinner: vegetable and tofu lasagna.
- Snack: oatmeal and raisin cookies
- Smoothie: Berry smoothie made with blueberries, strawberries, and soy milk

Day 13

- Breakfast: scrambled tofu with spinach and mushrooms.
- Lunch: roasted vegetables and hummus wrap.
- Dinner is mushroom and lentil shepherd's pie.
- Snack: Banana and oatmeal bars.
- Tropical smoothie made with pineapple, mango, and coconut water.

Day 14

- Breakfast: Coconut yogurt with granola and berries.
- Lunch: A black bean and corn quinoa bowl.
- Dinner: Thai green curry and rice.
- Snack: Date and Nut Balls
- Chocolate smoothie made with cocoa, banana, and oat milk.

CONCLUSION

As you reach the end of the "Plant-Based Gut Health Cookbook," I'd like to express my heartfelt gratitude for joining me on this nourishing journey. We've explored the rich tapestry of plant-based living, uncovering the secrets to a healthier, happier gut.

As we conclude this culinary adventure, I encourage you to incorporate these newfound insights and flavors into your daily life.

Consistency is essential on the path to optimal gut health. Consider incorporating a variety of plant-based dishes into your daily routine, experimenting with flavors and enjoying the nutritional benefits they provide. Whether it's a colorful salad for lunch or a hearty plant-based stew for dinner, each choice benefits your gut and, by extension, your overall health.

While this cookbook serves as a guide, it is critical to recognize your body's uniqueness and health requirements. Consult with healthcare professionals for personalized advice, especially if you have specific health concerns. They can provide personalized advice to ensure that your plant-based journey is in sync with your specific health goals.

I am so grateful for the opportunity to be a part of your health and wellness journey. If this cookbook has had a positive impact on your life, I would appreciate hearing from you. Your thoughts and experiences may encourage others to embark on their own plant-based journey. Please consider providing feedback, whether through a review.

Thank you for including me in a small part of your culinary journey. May your journey to vibrant gut health be filled with joy, delicious discoveries, and the profound satisfaction that comes from feeding your body plant-based goodness. Here's to your health, happiness, and ongoing celebration of life as you embrace a plant-based lifestyle.

I wish you a future full of vitality and wellbeing.